I0119779

Charles Higgens

Handbook of Ophthalmic Practice

Charles Higgens

Handbook of Ophthalmic Practice

ISBN/EAN: 9783337815479

Printed in Europe, USA, Canada, Australia, Japan

Cover: Foto ©Andreas Hilbeck / pixelio.de

More available books at **www.hansebooks.com**

OF

OPHTHALMIC PRACTICE.

BY

CHARLES HIGGINS, M.D., F.R.C.S.,
Assistant Surgeon and Lecturer in Ophthalmic Department,
Guy's Hospital.

SECOND EDITION, REVISED.

PHILADELPHIA:
P. BLAKISTON, SON & CO.,
1012 Walnut Street.
1882.

CONTENTS.

SECTION I.

SECTION II.

SECTION III.

SECTION IV.

SECTION V.

SECTION VI.

SECTION VII.

SECTION VIII.

OPHTHALMIC

OUT-PATIENT PRACTICE.

SECTION I.

DISCHARGE FROM THE EYES.

DISCHARGE from the eyes, in by far the greater number of cases in which it occurs, indicates inflammation of the conjunctiva—"Ophthalmia," as it is called. Patients suffering from ophthalmia present themselves complaining of smarting pain, and they state that the eyelids are gummed together on waking in the morning; the eyes are bloodshot, the lids may be red and more or less swollen, and there is more or less profuse mucous, muco-purulent, or purulent discharge.

We should examine the ocular conjunctiva, next draw down the lower lid so as to expose its conjunctival surface, then evert the upper lid, and carefully examine the conjunctiva covering it.

In order to evert the upper lid, whilst the patient is standing in front of us, we direct him to look downwards and close the eyes gently, then place the forefinger on the surface of the lid we wish to evert, press gently downwards and backwards, so as to make the free edge of the lid stand away from the eyeball, then place the thumb beneath the edge of the lid and lift it upwards, at the same time continuing the pressure with the forefinger; the tarsal cartilage is thus made to roll upon its long axis, and the lid becomes everted.

Should any difficulty be experienced in everting the lid—as is sometimes the case where there is thickening of the conjunctiva—we shall find that we can overcome it by using a probe in place of the forefinger. The probe should be pressed horizontally on the surface of the lid, whilst its margin is drawn upward by seizing the eyelashes between the finger and thumb of the disengaged hand.

The varieties of ophthalmia commonly met with are—Catarrhal (C. O.), Chronic (Ch. O.),

Granular (Gr. O.), Purulent (P. O.), and Phlyctenular (Pht. O.).*

Catarrhal Ophthalmia is characterized by rather profuse muco-purulent discharge, general injection, and sometimes swelling of the conjunctiva, with, in many cases, small blood extravasations in the substance of its ocular portion. As a rule both eyes are affected, the disease having commenced in one and spread to the other in the course of a day or two; it is acute in its course, and is highly contagious; we frequently see—amongst the out-patients—whole families affected.

Treatment.—In the early stage, if there be much pain and congestion, with only scanty discharge, we use fomentations of poppyheads: subsequently, when the discharge has become free, we order alum lotion—gr. vj to water ℥j—to be applied† to the eyes three, four, or six

---

* The letters in brackets are abbreviations.

† Alum lotion can be best applied by bathing, the eyes being partially opened during the application, so that some of the lotion gets between the lids. The ointment is only used to prevent the lids gumming together, and any simple ointment is equally as efficacious as that recommended.

times a day, or oftener, according to the severity of the attack; we prescribe the mild nitrate of mercury ointment—*i. e.*, one part of the ordinary ung. hyd. nitratis to eleven of lard—to be applied to the edges of the eyelids on going to bed.

Chronic Ophthalmia is often a sequel of the foregoing. It is characterized by injection of the palpebral conjunctiva, and some swelling of the semilunar fold and caruncle, the ocular conjunctiva being but little affected; the discharge is only slight, and consists principally of mucus, which collects in little masses at the inner canthi, and dries upon the margins of the lids, forming a scurf.

Treatment.—Alum lotion may be used, as in catarrhal ophthalmia, or we order guttæ zinci chlor.—gr. j or gr. ij of chloride of zinc to water ℥j—to be dropped into the eyes two or three times a day. It is, however, well to ring the changes between the chloride and sulphate of zinc, sulphate of copper, or other astringents, as after a time any single one loses its effect. We also order some ointment* to be applied to the

---

* Of late the ointments employed in the ophthalmic department have been made with vaseline instead of lard.

edges of the eyelids at bedtime, to prevent their gumming together.

Granular Ophthalmia is a much more serious affection than either of the foregoing. The usual symptoms of ophthalmia are present, and besides the patient often complains of a feeling of roughness about the eyelids; there may be much pain, and intolerance of light; the lids may be thickened, the cornea may be more or less opaque and vascular, the condition known as "pannus" having been developed. The lids may be distorted, giving rise to inversion of their margins—"entropion;" or some of the eyelashes may be misdirected, and turn inwards —"trichiasis." On exposing the palpebral conjunctiva by eversion of the lids, we find it rough and vascular, and covered more or less thickly with granular bodies of various sizes and shapes, or perhaps deeply scarred, ridged, and furrowed,

---

Many of them have to be kept for considerable periods, and the lard frequently decomposes, whilst vaseline will keep in exactly the same condition for any length of time. The application of drops should be made by drawing down the lower lid, and applying a small quantity of the solution to its conjunctival surface, with either a quill or camel's-hair pencil.

all trace of the healthy membrane having disappeared. We notice that the changes in the conjunctiva are most marked about the attached or upper border of the superior tarsal cartilage. The condition in which we find the conjunctiva varies with the length of time the disease has existed; in early cases we find red, or pale, granular bodies; in later ones the scarred, ridged, and furrowed appearance already alluded to.

Treatment.—Granular ophthalmia is of all ophthalmic diseases perhaps the most rebellious to treatment. In the more acute cases we apply the mitigated nitrate of silver stick—nitrate of silver, one part to three of nitrate of potash—twice a week, or oftener; in the older cases we use the lapis divinus, or green stone, as often as may appear necessary.* The green stone

* The application of the mitigated nitrate of silver stick or green stone should be made as follows:—Having placed the patient in a chair, we stand behind him, rest his head firmly against our chest, then evert the lids, and brush the whole of the palpebral conjunctiva thoroughly over with mitigated stick or green stone; if the former be used, we wash the conjunctiva with salt and water (gr. xx to ℥j) before allowing the lids to return to their natural position.

is made of alum, sulphate of copper, nitrate of potash, and camphor (*vide* Guy's "Pharmacopœia").

In most cases we order sulphate of copper drops—sulphate of copper gr. ij, water ℥j—to be used three or four times daily, and some of the mild nitrate, or other ointment, to be applied to the edges of the lids at night. In those cases, however, in which there is much intolerance of light, or in which we suspect that iritis is present, as sometimes happens, we order atropine drops—sulphate of atropine gr. j, water ℥j—to be used instead of the sulphate of copper drops; or an ointment—gr. ¼ of sulphate of atropine, gr. ¼ of acetate of morphia, to ʒj of vaseline—may be employed; a small portion of the ointment should be placed on the inner surface of the lower eyelids two or three times a day. If "entropion" exist we remedy it by operation; inverted lashes, if only few in number, we remove with cilia forceps; but should a quantity turn inwards, we must remove the hair bulbs and tissue in which they rest with the knife. Cases of granular ophthalmia of long standing are rarely permanently cured, but the disease can be kept in check by careful and persevering treatment. There are now amongst the out-patients many who have been attending more or less regularly for years. Slight cases should be cured in the course of three to six months, if persevered with.

Purulent Ophthalmia is of all inflammations of the conjunctiva the most severe, and the most likely to give rise to permanent impairment, or complete loss, of vision, by causing ulceration or sloughing of the cornea.

The most violent form of purulent ophthalmia is that occasioned by inoculation with gonorrhœal matter—it is known as "gonorrhœal ophthalmia;" we must, however, bear in mind that by no means all cases of purulent ophthalmia have this origin.

In the early stage of purulent ophthalmia there is no sign by which we can distinguish it from catarrhal ophthalmia; and, indeed, mild cases of the former and severe cases of the latter are scarcely to be distinguished.

In the more severe forms, however, the lids soon become greatly swollen, so as to nearly or quite close the eyes; copious purulent discharge issues from between them; we find the ocular conjunctiva intensely red and much swollen, constituting what is known as "chemosis;" the palpebral conjunctiva is also swollen and vascular, the fold between the lower lid and globe (fornix) in some cases protruding from the palpebral aperture: there is severe pain, and often considerable constitutional disturbance.

Purulent ophthalmia may occur in newly-born children, or in older persons; in the former it is known as "ophthalmia neonatorum." Ophthalmia neonatorum may arise from contact of acrid vaginal secretions during parturition, or from dirt and exposure after birth; the most severe form is that caused by contact or gonorrhœal pus. Purulent ophthalmia in older persons may arise from contact with pus from a similar case, or from inoculation with gonorrhœal matter. Whether the disease occurs in infants or other patients, both eyes are frequently affected; but should it exist in one only, we must carefully cover the other with pad, strapping, and a bandage, so as if possible to prevent it becoming inoculated.

In every case of purulent ophthalmia we should carefully examine the cornea, as upon its condition our prognosis, with regard to sight, must be based. If the cornea be clear our prognosis is favorable, but if hazy, ulcerated, or perforated, more or less impairment of vision will result; we must always use the greatest gentleness in making our examination, as a threatening perforation may be made complete by rough handling.

Treatment.—In cases of "ophthalmia neonatorum" we order the eyes to be syringed out with alum lotion so often as the discharge collects; every hour, half hour, or even more frequently, if necessary; time should, however, be allowed at night for sleep; we order some simple ointment to be smeared on the edges and surfaces of the lids—so as to keep them constantly greasy—and direct the greatest cleanliness to be observed. The treatment must be steadily persevered in until the discharge becomes sensibly diminished in quantity, and altered in quality, and may be gradually left off as improvement takes place.

In mild cases of purulent ophthalmia in older persons, the frequent use of alum lotion with some ointment smeared on the edges of the eyelids at bedtime will suffice for a cure; but in the severer forms, and especially in "gonorrhœal ophthalmia," we must have recourse to much more energetic treatment.

At the patient's first visit the conjunctiva should be carefully brushed over with solid nitrate of silver, and then washed with salt and water. We should apply four, five, or more leeches to the temples, order the eyes to be constantly bathed with alum lotion, grs. x to ℥j of water; the lotion may with advantage be iced, and a bag of ice laid upon the closed lids during the intervals at which the lotion is applied; a good purge should be administered at first, but when the bowels have been well cleared out; quinine, or iron, or both, should be prescribed with liberal diet, and a fair amount of stimulant. As already stated, the danger in purulent ophthalmia is damage to the cornea, and the more vigorous the state of health of our patient the less likely is this to occur. We must give opium at night in cases in which much pain is complained of.

In any case of purulent ophthalmia, if we find the cornea ulcerated, we must support it by the application of a good pad and bandage; by this means we may often save perforation; the bandage must, however, be frequently removed in order to apply the alum lotion, with which the pad should also be kept wetted.

Phlyctenular Ophthalmia is characterized by the existence of small patches of vascularity, usually situated near the corneal margin.

On examination these vascular patches are found to be associated with small pale elevations of varying size and number, there being in some cases only two or three large ones, in others several of smaller size; there is some watering of the eye and some slight mucous discharge; there may be some intolerance of light.

Treatment.—We dust some calomel into the eye at the patient's visit, and order the yellow oxide of mercury ointment (yellow oxide of mercury gr. ij to iv, vaseline ʒj), a small portion to be placed on the inner surface of the lower eyelid at bedtime; we also prescribe tonics should the condition of the patient indicate their use.

SECTION II.

INTOLERANCE OF LIGHT.

(*Photophobia.*)

A PATIENT—most frequently a child—presents himself or is brought suffering from "intolerance of light," the intolerance being often associated with very profuse lachrymation, and at times with some mucous discharge.

In all cases in which intolerance of light is a prominent symptom, we should suspect, and shall generally find, corneal disease.

In any case we make a careful examination of the surface of the cornea. Adults and children of fair age can usually be persuaded to open the eyes themselves, if we take care to shade them from too bright light. In little children the lids are often so tightly screwed up that we have to open them by force.

We find the easiest method of making an

examination in such cases is, whilst sitting in a chair opposite to the nurse, who firmly holds the child's legs, arms, and body, we fix its head firmly between our knees; we can thus hold it as still as if fixed in a vice. We then place the forefinger of one hand on the margin of the upper lid, and press it firmly but gently upwards and backwards beneath the margin of the orbit; then with the thumb of the other hand we draw down the lower lid. A good view of the cornea is thus obtained.

The diseases most frequently met with are (1) *Corneal ulcers.* In these cases there is evident loss of substance of the corneal surface; the ulcers vary in number, depth, and position; at times they are opaque, and have considerable vascularity about them, at others they are transparent, and present no signs of bloodvessels. (2) Some form of *Corneitis*—(A) *Pustular* or *phlyctenular corneitis* most frequently met with in children, and very much the same disease as phlyctenular ophthalmia, with this difference, that the phlyctenulæ are developed on the corneal surface, and are generally smaller and in greater numbers. The phlyctenulæ have often degenerated into pustules or ulcers. Pustular corneitis, occurring in strumous, unhealthy children, is often described as a separate disease, under the name of strumous corneitis. *Strumous corneitis* is characterized by great intolerance of light, often out of all proportion to any visible disease. On examination small ulcers, surrounded by a halo of dullness, are found on the cornea; they have a bundle of vessels leading to them, and are at times described as vascular ulcers. The eyelids are frequently much swollen, and may be covered by eczematous eruptions; the child may also be suffering from eczema capitis. (B) *Interstitial* or *parenchymatous keratitis* (*syphilitic keratitis*, or *corneitis*, *corneo-iritis*, *diffuse keratitis*, *diffuse vascular keratitis*). This disease is met with in children and young adults, and is frequently, but by no means always, associated with the peculiar physiognomy of congenital syphilis, notched or malformed teeth, &c. It affects one eye first, the other nearly always following. It is marked by gradually increasing haziness, commencing at the centre of the cornea; the haze gradually spreads; at parts small bloodvessels are developed, giving rise to a peculiar brick-dust color, quite characteristic of this form of inflammation; the inflammation may continue until the whole cornea has the appearance of a piece of ground glass of a reddish color, or it may stop at any stage short of this; in any case much greater clearing of the corneal tissues takes place than might be expected. Intolerance of light is a rather variable symptom, but occurs in most cases, and in some is very severe. The corneal inflammation is not unfrequently associated with iritis. We should always warn the patient that the disease is sure to last at least six months, and very possibly longer, and having decided on any plan of treatment, persevere with it. (c) *Pannus* (already mentioned under granular ophthalmia). In this disease the cornea is found more or less fleshy and vascular. The position of the vessels must be carefully noted. Should they commence in the conjunctiva covering the sclerotic, pass over the margin of the cornea, and traverse its surface, the case is one of "pannus." But should the vessels appear to commence in the cornea near its margin, and lie wholly within its area, the case is one of corneitis—most probably interstitial. We must pay special attention to these points, as the treatment of the two diseases differs widely.

Pannus is caused by friction. When it exists we examine the palpebral conjunctiva, and shall very probably find some form of granulation. Should the conjunctiva appear healthy, we examine the margins of the lids. Some few lashes may be found growing inwards and irritating the cornea, or the whole row in the upper or lower lid may be found misdirected. (*See* Sec. I.) (D) Suppurative corneitis; this not unfrequently follows blows upon the cornea. We find a collection of pus in the substance of the cornea, some of which has probably escaped into the anterior chamber; there is severe pain and great photophobia.

(3) Foreign bodies, on the surface of the cornea, in its substance, or adhering to the conjunctival surface of the lids, or injuries to the cornea, may all give rise to intolerance of light. (*See* Sec. VIII.)

Treatment.—Corneal ulcers, pustular corneitis, and strumous corneitis, are best treated locally by keeping the eyes carefully bandaged with lint soaked in belladonna lotion;* by frequently bathing the eyes with belladonna lotion; and by

---

* Extract of belladonna gr. vj to gr. x, water ℥j.

the occasional instillation of solution of sulphate of atropine,* gr. iv to ℥j. Some cases, however, do best with the yellow oxide of mercury ointment applied in the same manner as for phlyctenular ophthalmia; it must be used with caution, and discontinued if it cause much pain and irritation without any very marked improvement. Constitutionally, by the administration of tonics, as steel wine, dialysed iron, or perchloride of iron, with cod liver oil. We should also, especially in children, direct that wholesome, nourishing food is given; the appetites of these little patients are often extremely capricious, and are satisfied with sweets, pastry, &c. Specific keratitis in young children is best treated locally in the same manner, but we shall find that the internal administration of grey powder in doses of gr. j to iij does good in many cases. In older persons we should order guttæ atropiæ (gr. ½ to gr. ij of sulphate of atropine to ℥j of water) to be dropped into the eyes

* We should always be careful, in prescribing atropine, to order the *sulphate*, and direct the solution to be made from the crystals dissolved in distilled water alone, otherwise the liquor atropinæ—which contains spirit, and causes great irritation if dropped into the eye—may be given.

three to twelve times a day, according to the severity of the attack; give mercurials in the earlier stages of the disease, followed by tonics in the later.

In cases of corneal disease, should there be much discharge, we should order alum or some other astringent to be mixed with the belladonna lotion or atropine drops. Suppurative corneitis is best treated by warm applications; the eye should be bathed frequently with hot belladonna lotion, and kept carefully bandaged with pads of lint soaked in the lotion. If perforation appear imminent, the pus must be let out by an incision passing through the whole thickness of the cornea, or iridectomy must be performed.

The pain must be relieved by opium internally, and application of leeches (2 to 6) to the temple; good diet must be ordered, and iron or quinine given.

The treatment of "pannus" depends upon its cause. Should it be caused by granular lids, we must treat the granulations (*see* Sect. I); inverted lashes, or other sources of irritation, must be removed; we should, however, order atropine to be used frequently in addition to the other treatment.

The eczematous eruptions so frequently met with in children suffering from corneal disease are best treated locally by great attention to cleanliness, and by the application of ung. hydr. ammoniat., either alone or mixed with sulphur ointment in equal parts.

Lotions containing lead must be avoided in ophthalmic practice; they are very useful in some forms of conjunctival inflammation, but should there be ulceration of the cornea, a deposit of carbonate of lead will very probably form upon its surface, giving rise to a dense white opacity.

In some cases of corneal disease, associated with obstinate intolerance of light, the insertion of setons in the temples often acts like magic in removing the photophobia.

SECTION III.

IRITIS AND GLAUCOMA.

Iritis.

A PATIENT presents himself complaining of some watering of the eye, some impairment of vision, and perhaps some intolerance of light or pain, as a rule one eye only being affected.

On examination we find in all cases some cloudiness and loss of polish of the iris, sluggishness or immobility of the—as a rule—contracted pupil, and injection in the ciliary region.* In some cases we may find considerable col-

* The ciliary region comprises a portion of the ocular tissues contained in a zone, immediately surrounding the cornea, and corresponding to the situation of the ciliary body. The vessels of the ciliary region which lie beneath the conjunctiva, in the sub-conjunctival fascia, always become more or less gorged with blood in inflammations of the cornea or iris, and often in those of the chlorid or ciliary body, so that in all cases of iritis, as also in corneitis, and in many cases of choroiditis, &c., we shall find a more or less distinct vascular zone surrounding the cornea.

lections of lymph, either in nodules or diffused evenly over the surface of the iris, irregularity of the pupil, blocking of its area by inflammatory material, adhesions of its margin to the lens capsule, "posterior synechiæ;" or suppuration may have taken place, giving rise to collection of pus in the anterior chamber—"hypopyon;" or abscess in the substances of the iris. The presence of nodules of lymph upon the iris shows that the iritis is syphilitic. The lymph nodules are, however, rarely present, and there is no other sign by which we can distinguish iritis dependent on syphilis from that which arise from other causes; so that if we wish to ascertain the nature of an iritis we shall have to go upon other data than those presented by the appearance of the affected eye.

In severe cases iritis is easily recognized; but it is of the greatest importance that we should detect it in its slight or incipient forms.

It is in the early stage of iritis that well-directed treatment is most likely to be successful in preventing the adhesions of the iris to the lens capsule, and the formation of opacities in the pupil, which so frequently occur, and which are so frequently the cause of permanent impairment of vision. Pain is a most variable and uncertain symptom in iritis; in many cases it is entirely absent, in some it may be slight, whilst in others it is extremely severe. Iritis is very liable to be overlooked should it set in in the course of ophthalmia, or inflammation of other structures of the globe. If we are in doubt, the behavior of the pupil on the instillation of atropine will as a rule clear it up. Should iritis be present, the pupil, instead of becoming large and circular will dilate irregularly, or not at all. It may be laid down as an axiom in ophthalmic practice, *when in doubt use atropine.* The cases in which it can do harm are rare, whilst those in which it will do good are innumerable.

Treatment.—Our first care should be, if possible, *to dilate the pupil;* to this end we apply to the conjunctiva a solution of sulphate of atropine, gr. iv to ℥j, at the time of our patient's visit, and prescribe for him a solution of gr. j to ℥j to use himself three or four times a day. If at the next visit the pupil still remains contracted, we apply more of the strong solution, and order the weaker one to be used more frequently (six or twelve times a day). So soon as the pupil begins to dilate we have gone a great way toward the cure of iritis.

In some cases atropine causes a kind of erysipelatous inflammation of the skin of the eyelids and cheeks; the condition is known as "atropism." Should atropism occur, we must order some kind of ointment to be smeared over the affected parts, fomentations of poppyheads to be used frequently, and discontinue the use of atropine.

As soon as the inflammation has subsided we must find some substitute for the atropine solutions. Solutions of daturine, sulphate of hyoscyamine, or duboisin, may be tried, or we give an ointment consisting of gr. ½ of sulphate of atropine, gr. ½ of acetate of morphia to ʒj of vaseline, a small portion to be placed on the conjunctival surface of the lower eyelid three times a day. In slight cases of iritis only local treatment to the eye itself is needed; in more severe ones especially if associated with severe pain, we order two to six leeches to be applied to the temple, and give opium if necessary. In cases where a large quantity of inflammatory material is thrown out, we give mercury so as just to affect the gums, and we may lay it down as a rule, which seldom needs to be departed from, *that lymph upon the iris calls for the ad-*

ministration of mercury; we need not trouble ourselves to ascertain whether or no the iritis be syphilitic.

In suppurative iritis we give tonics, the perchloride of iron being as good as any; and, instead of using atropine, order the eye to be bathed frequently with hot belladonna lotion, and kept bandaged in the intervals with a pad of lint soaked in the lotion laid over the closed lids.

Glaucoma.

Speaking broadly, glaucoma is a disease characterized by *increase of tension of the eyeball,* to which may be referred most of the other symptoms met with. It as a rule attacks persons beyond middle age, and affects both eyes, though often at considerable intervals. We divide the disease into simple, acute, chronic, and secondary glaucoma.

In simple glaucoma, complaints are made of very gradually increasing impairment of vision, occasional obscurations of the visual field by a yellow smoky cloud, appearance of a halo around a flame, at times colored like a rainbow, and that glasses which first assisted vision have soon to be changed for stronger ones; no pain is experienced. On examination, we find slight increase of tension* of one or both eyes, some dilatation of the pupil, with great sluggishness of its movements, a hazy appearance of the lens and contraction of the visual field, though central vision may be acute; there are no inflammatory symptoms. We may find engorgement of the veins emerging from sclerotic in the ciliary region.

The ophthalmoscope shows venous hyperæmia of the retina, pulsation of the retinal arteries, either spontaneous or easily produced by pressure on the eyeball, and very probably cupping of the optic disc;† if the disease have lasted

---

* We ascertain the tension of eyeballs thus:—Direct the patient to look downwards and gently close the eyes, then with a finger of each hand we make gentle alternate pressure upon the globe through the closed upper lid, in the same manner as we should do if ascertaining the existence of fluctuation in any other part. In the normal state, the eyeball is firm and semi-elastic, its tension may vary either on the side of increase or decrease. We express the degree of tension by nine T's, thus:—If tension is normal as Tn, if above par as T+1, T+2, T+3; if below par, as T—1, T—2, T—3; if a doubt exists, as T+? or T—?

† The cupped optic disc is characterized by a bluish appearance of its central part, which is surrounded by a

long, atrophy of the disc will have commenced; we may meet with retinal hæmorrhages. The hazy appearance of the lens, coupled with the gradual impairment of vision often leads to the very fatal error of mistaking *simple glaucoma for cataract.* The ophthalmoscope will, however, always save us from making such a blunder; an examination will show us that the opacity is more apparent than real, and that we can obtain a clear view of the fundus upon which we shall find some of the changes already mentioned.

It is of the greatest importance that simple glaucoma should not be confounded with cataract; the mistake is often made, and the patient, whose vision might have been saved by a timely iridectomy, allowed to become irremediably blind, whilst waiting for the supposed cataract to become mature.

Acute and chronic glaucoma are marked by

---

very distinct whiteish rim; the retinal vessels appear thin upon the blue part of the disc; as they get up to the margin their course appears broken, and they reappear upon the retina dilated and tortuous, at a point not continuous with the former direction.

Pulsation is seen as an alternate emptying and filling of the vessels.

more or less severe inflammatory attacks, and hence are sometimes described as "inflammatory glaucoma." Both are usually preceded by a premonitory stage, resembling in great measure simple glaucoma, but differing from it in that sooner or later an inflammatory outbreak occurs; this never happens in simple glaucoma, which goes gradually on till vision is entirely extinguished without a single attack of inflammation or pain.

A patient attacked by acute glaucoma, after having passed through a premonitory stage, usually of only short duration, is suddenly attacked often in the night by severe pain, accompanied by marked inflammatory symptoms; the pain is often agonizing, and affects not only the eye but the whole of the corresponding side of the head; there may be considerable constitutional disturbance, and not unfrequently nausea and vomiting; should the patient attempt to see with the affected eye, he will find vision reduced to perception of light. On examination we find the eyelids swollen, the conjuctiva congested, and the vascularity of the eyeball generally increased; *the globe is stony hard* (T+3), the cornea looks steamy, the aqueous is cloudy, the anterior chamber shallower than normal, the iris discolored, the pupil *dilated* and fixed, the lens hazy-looking. The ophthalmoscope shows the vitreous to be hazy, so that no details of the fundus can be clearly made out, though we may see the optic disc indistinctly.

There are certain symptoms in acute glaucoma which may mislead; thus I have seen the nausea and vomiting lead to the diagnosis of biliousness, the pain has been put down to neuralgia, the swelling of the lids to erysipelas; the patient has been treated in accordance with these views, the ocular symptoms being overlooked, until irremediable blindness has set in. It is worthy of note that acute glaucoma very frequently comes on in persons laid up and suffering from other diseases or accidents. Thus, I have seen it in a case of carbuncle, in one of abscess, in another of fractured ankle; in each of these the glaucoma was neither diagnosed nor treated. An attack of acute glaucoma may pass off, leaving the eye harder than normal, and with vision more or less impaired. This period of "*remission*" may last for some time, but sooner or later another attack comes on, which may again subside, but only to be followed by others, which will if not prevented, inevitably destroy vision.

We do not find cupping of the disc in acute glaucoma; the cup takes time to develop, and the course of acute glaucoma is so rapid that before the excavation takes place vision is lost, and the media become too hazy to allow of a view of the fundus being obtained.

Chronic glaucoma is marked by a longer premonitory stage than the acute; the inflammatory attacks are well-marked, but are much less violent, occur at longer intervals, and subside without leaving so great impairment of vision; the pain is much less severe; cupping of the optic disc becomes well-marked; the retinal veins become gorged; pulsation of the retinal arteries is seen; in fact, chronic glaucoma may be looked upon as simple glaucoma plus attacks of inflammation and pain; the tension of the globe is, however, greater, and as a consequence the morbid changes are more marked and rapid.

By secondary glaucoma we mean glaucoma coming on in the course of some other ocular affection—thus, we may meet with it in cases of corneitis, wounds or perforations of the cornea causing anterior synechia; injuries to the lens, displacing it, or causing it to become opaque and swell; in some affections of the choroid iris, or retina, etc. This form may attack patients of any age.

Both the acute and chronic forms of glaucoma have been mistaken for iritis; we shall avoid such an error by attending—1st, to the condition of the pupil—in glaucoma it is dilated, in iritis almost invariably contracted; 2d, the tension of the globe is always *considerably* increased in inflammatory glaucoma, in iritis it is normal, or perhaps *very slightly* above par. Inflammatory glaucoma resembles iritis in that there is injection of the ciliary region, dimness of vision, more or less immobility of the pupil and discoloration of the iris. We must avoid the use of atropine in glaucoma, as it may increase the tension and do great harm. *Glaucoma can only be cured by operation.*

So soon as the nature of the disease is manifest we must perform iridectomy; the earlier the operation is done the greater is our chance of success; to wait is simply to lose valuable time and lessen the chance of restoration of vision.

Iridectomy (how, we do not know) reduces the tension of the eyeball. That the operation may be effectual we must take care *to remove the iris quite down to its greater circumference, and excise a good broad piece.* Should the first operation fail, a second or even third should be performed. We must do our best to impress upon our patient the necessity for an early operation, and should we fail in gaining his consent the sooner we allow him to seek other advice the better for our credit.

SECTION IV.

DISEASES OF THE EYELIDS.

The most frequently met with diseases of the eyelids are—

Tinea (not a parasitic disease, described also under the names of "ophthalmia tarsi and blepharitis,") a chronic ulcerative inflammation in and around the follicles of the eye-lashes. We find crusts of exudation adhering to the margins of the lids amongst the lashes; the exudation may form only a slight scurf, or there may be a quantity of dense brownish-yellow scabs. On removing the scabs we find the margin of the lid fissured and bleeding. In old cases the lids may become much thickened, the lower ones being everted, and giving rise to displacement of the tear puncta, in consequence of which the tears constantly flow over and irritate the skin of the lids and cheek. The sufferers are usually children.

Treatment.—Tinea in its more severe forms is very rebellious to treatment. Slight cases can be cured in a few weeks, by great attention to cleanliness, the application of the mild nitrate of mercury ointment to the margins of the lids (from which all exudation has been carefully washed away*) at night, and bathing with alum lotion three or four times a day.

In severe cases (in addition to the use of the lotion and ointment) the eye-lashes should be picked out with forceps, the scales removed, and the raw services left touched with a point of solid nitrate of silver; one application will usually be sufficient.

Should the lower tear puncta be displaced, we must slit the punctum and canaliculus in each lower lid (*see* Sec. V.) Any constitutional treatment which may appear necessary should be employed.

Hordeolum, or stye, is met with as a red, inflamed, painful, and usually suppurating swelling, near the margin of the lid. Styes often come in successive crops; they show a debilitated state of health. We order poultices at night, and fomentations during the day; as

* The exudation can be washed away with soda and warm water. Should any scales appear particularly tenacious, they should be picked off with the nail.

soon as the pus begins to point the little swelling should be opened. The tincture of perchloride of iron in doses of from five to twenty minims, according to the age of the patient, is the best internal remedy.

Tarsal Cyst somewhat resembles hordeolum in appearance; it is, however, usually situated further from the margin of the lid, and is but seldom inflamed, painful, or suppurating. On everting the lid, a purple spot will be seen marking its position on the conjunctival surface.

Tarsal cyst is caused by an obstruction of the duct of a Meibomian gland, the retained secretion of which forms a tumor.

Treatment.—We puncture the cyst through the purple spot on the conjunctival surface, scarify its interior thoroughly with the point of the knife, and scoop out the contents with a spoon-ended probe, or squeeze them out between the fingers. The contents of the cyst usually consist of a jelly-like material, but occasionally suppuration has taken place and the cyst is filled with pus, in which case it is sufficient to lay it open and leave the pus to escape of itself.

When the contents have been evacuated, the cyst will fill with blood, and the tumor will be as large, or larger, than before it was opened; we should warn our patient of this. The blood will absorb in the course of a few weeks, when the tumor will disappear; should it remain of any size at the end of five or six weeks, the cyst must be opened afresh.

Molluscum is a small whiteish tumor, having a depression in its centre; we frequently meet with one or several of the little growths upon the skin of the eyelid and face; they should be freely incised, and their contents—which are of a cheesy nature—squeezed out between the thumb-nails.

Warts are occasionally met with about the eyelids; they should be cut off with scissors.

SECTION V.

WATERING OF THE EYE.

WATERING of the eye, "epiphora,"* occurs as the result of hypersecretion in many of the inflammatory affections of the eye, and may result from displacement of the tear puncta (*see* Sec. IV), but should it occur alone, or accompanied by muco-purulent discharge, obstruction of the tear passages is indicated. The obstruction may be at the tear punctum, in the canaliculus, or at its entrance into the lachrymal sac, or in the lachrymal duct; the most common situation being at the junction of the duct with the sac, and next to this at the exit of the duct into the inferior meatus of the nose.

Should the obstruction be in either of the

* The term epiphora is sometimes confined to cases where the watering is due to over-secretion; whilst that of "stillicidium" lachrymarum is applied in cases where the overflow is due to obstruction of the tear passages. We will, however, be content with the one term—epiphora.

three first situations, epiphora will be the only symptom; but if in either of the last, we shall have, in addition to the watering, more or less distension of the lachrymal sac, forming a tumor at the side of the nose.

Pressure upon the tumor will cause its subsidence, with the escape through the tear puncta —of (1) thick tenacious transparent mucus, (2) the same turbid from mixture with pus, or (3) pus itself.

Treatment.—In any cases of epiphora, whether simple or associated with discharge, we first make a fair trial of astringent lotions applied to the inner canthus, so that they may find their way into the tear passages.*

These failing to do good, we should slit up the tear punctum and canaliculus of the lower lid (the upper canaliculus seldom requires to be meddled with). Should the obstruction be situated at the punctum, or in the canaliculus, we shall thus entirely cure the epiphora, and may greatly improve some cases in which the obstruction is lower down. Opening the canaliculus gives free exit to pent-up secretion in

* The same lotions as those recommended for ophthalmia should be used.

the sac, and its mucous membrane takes on a more healthy action.

In any case, after having slit the canaliculus—even if no improvement take place—we should abstain from further operative interference for five or six weeks. We merely take care that the slit canaliculus does not close, that the sac is kept empty by pressure with the finger whenever it begins to fill, and that astringent lotions are used constantly. At the end of the time specified we must try to relieve the structure of the duct by passing probes.

Slitting the Lower Tear Punctum and Canaliculus. We place the patient in a chair, stand behind him and rest his head, over which a towel has been thrown, against the lower part of our chest; then, supposing the right side to be operated on, place the small and third fingers of the left hand upon the patient's face near the outer canthus, draw the lids tense with these two fingers and keep them so; next take the small-grooved director in the right hand and pass it at first vertically through the punctum, then depress its handle and pass it horizontally along the canaliculus into the sac; to be certain that the director is in the sac, we relax the tension kept up by the two fingers of the left hand and push the director gently with the right; should there be any puckering-up at the inner canthus when the director is thus pushed, it has not entered the sac, and a further attempt must be made; if no puckering be caused, we bring the lids again into a state of tension as before, transfer the handle of the director to the thumb and forefinger of the same hand, and then take in the right hand a common cataract or any other small knife that will cut and run it along the groove in the director well into the sac; the upper lid must be kept out of the way by one of the fingers of the right hand. The left side is operated on in the same manner, excepting that the hands are reversed. The upper canaliculus sometimes requires slitting; the operation is not quite so simple as that on the lower. The patient must be seen daily for the next three days, and the director passed along the slit to prevent its closing. To pass a probe down the nasal duct the position of the patient and operator are the same as for slitting the canaliculus. The canaliculus should have been slit at some previous time, the lids being made tense in the manner already described, the probe should be passed along the slit as far as it will go, the absence of puckering at the inner canthus on relaxation of the tension of the eyelids shows that the end of the probe is in the sac; being satisfied that the probe is in the sac, we raise it along the margin of the orbit (taking care all the time to keep the end firmly pressed against the inner wall of the sac) until it has attained a vertical position, then push it gently downwards and slightly backwards in the direction of the lachrymal duct; having passed the probe down the duct, we withdraw it a little, so as to raise its end off the floor of the nose, and leave it for some twenty minutes or longer. If the probe has been properly passed down the duct, its upper extremity will remain firmly fixed against the upper margin of the orbit. If the upper extremity moves freely about, it shows that the wall of the duct has been perforated, in which case the probe must be withdrawn and passed afresh.

The lachrymal sac not unfrequently becomes inflamed and suppurates.

In addition to "epiphora," we find a dusky-red and exquisitely painful swelling, situated at the side of the nose, the eyelids in their whole extent being more or less œdematous; should pus have formed, the swelling is tense and deeply fluctuating; as a rule, one side only is affected. The disease is sometimes mistaken for erysipelas, more especially should both sacs happen to be inflamed.

Treatment.—A free incision should be made through the skin into the sac, the earlier the better; poultices should be employed, and the general health attended to. When the inflammation has subsided, obstruction of the lachrymal duct—which is almost certain to exist—should be treated.

SECTION VI.

ACUTENESS OF VISION—FIELD OF VISION—ANOMALIES OF REFRACTION—ASTIGMATISM—RANGE OF ACCOMMODATION—PRESBYOPIA.

By acuteness of vision ($= v$) we understand the power which the eye possesses of distinguishing objects; we judge of the acuteness of vision by the use of letters of certain proportions, known as test types.

The test types we use are those of Dr. Snellen. The letters of these types are of such dimensions that they can be recognized by a fairly sharp-sighted eye at certain distances; the distance at which each set of letters should be recognized is marked over it. If the eye, the acuteness of vision of which we wish to ascertain, can recognize *any* of the letters at their proper distances, we assume that its acuteness of vision is normal.

We are, however, often met by a difficulty here, as we naturally suppose that an eye which can read one set of types at its proper distance should be able to recognize the rest also at their proper distances. Such, however, is not the case. We frequently find that an eye reads easily the types which should be recognized at a short distance, but makes out nothing of those which should be recognized at greater distances; and, on the contrary, that an eye of which the acuteness of vision for distance is normal, can with difficulty or not at all make out the types which should be recognized close to.

This apparent inconsistence, however, need not surprise us; it depends on what are known as anomalies of refraction (*see* p. 55 *et seq.*), and we shall find that on neutralizing these anomalies by suitable glasses, all the types will be recognized at their proper distances. We may express the acuteness of vision by the formula $v = \frac{d}{D}$, in which d = a certain distance—*e. g.*, 6 metres*—D the letters that can be read by

* In the new editions of Snellen's types the metrical system of measurement has been introduced, so that the distances of the types, instead of being measured in feet and inches as heretofore, are measured by metres and fractions of metres. The size of some of the letters has also been somewhat altered.

If we wish to use the old measurement, we have only to remember that a metre equals about 40 inches (39.4), so the eye we wish to examine at 6 metres; if *d* and D be the same, *i. e.*, if D = 6* can be read at 6 metres, the formula will be $v = \frac{6}{6}$ or 1, that is normal acuteness of vision; if D = 12 only can be made out at 6 metres, the formula will be $v = \frac{6}{12} = \frac{1}{2}$, and so on.

By field of vision we understand the area over which objects situated in the same vertical plane can be distinguished, the eye being meanwhile fixed. The field is limited by a line joining the most eccentrically placed points of objects that can thus be made out. We can ascertain the extent of the field of vision thus:—

We place our patient in a convenient position, stand opposite to him at a distance of about two feet, and, supposing we wish to examine his left eye, direct him to look steadily at our own right eye. The patient's right eye and our own left should be kept closed. We then move our hand

---

that it is very easy to alter the metrical measurement to our own; thus, the largest letter in the book of types, which used to be marked CC (200 feet) is now sixty, meaning sixty metres; but sixty metres equal 200 feet (nearly). XX is now six (six metres).

* See Snellen's Book of Types, which can be obtained from Messrs. Williams & Norgate, 14 Henrietta Street, Covent Garden.

in various directions in the peripheral parts of the field, and notice if its movements are perceived by the patient's eye at the same distance from the centre as by our own presumably healthy retina.

We must take care to move the hand in a vertical plane, situated midway between our own and the patient's eye, and also see that he keeps his eye fixed.

Should the eye under examination distinguish all movements of the hand at the same distance from the centre as our own, we decide that the field of vision is normal; but should a falling-off be noticed in any particular direction, we infer that the sensibility of the corresponding portion of retina is impaired.

It must be remembered that each part of the visual field corresponds to a portion of retina opposite to, and not on the same side as, the object seen, so that the outer half of the field belongs to the inner half of the retina, and *vice versa*. Limitation or contraction of the visual field is a very constant accompaniment of retinal charges, whether induced by the pressure of increased tension, as in glaucoma, or by disease of the retina itself, or of the optic nerve.

Anomalies of Refraction.

By refraction of the eyeball we understand its condition with reference to the formation of images of distant objects, the rays of light proceeding from which are assumed to be parallel; and this in a state of relaxation of its accommodation.

By accommodation we understand the power possessed by the eye of so altering the condition of *its refraction* as to adjust itself for diverging rays of light, or those proceeding from near objects.

An eye of normal refraction has an antero-posterior axis of such a length that parallel rays of light are brought to a focus exactly in the layer of rods and cones; such an eye is said to be "emmetropic."

An eye of abnormal refraction may have an antero-posterior axis, either too long or too short; such eyes are said to be "ametropic." *We see that the refraction depends upon the length of the eyeball.*

The eye of too long antero-posterior axis is called "myopic;" that of too short antero-posterior axis "hypermetropic;" these two conditions constitute what are known as anomalies of refraction, or "myopia and hypermetropia." We can diagnose anomalies of refraction by trial with lenses, and by direct ophthalmoscopic examination.

In order to diagnose anomalies of refraction by trial with lenses, we must be provided with Snellen's test types, already alluded to, and with a box of trial glasses.

The lenses we now use are numbered in what are known as "dioptrics," a "dioptric" = D, being a lens of 1 metre focus; a lens of two dioptrics is double the strength of that of one dioptric, and has a focal length of half a metre (50 centimetres); a lens of three dioptrics is three times as strong as a lens of one dioptric, and has a focal length one-third of a metre (about 33 centimetres).

A Table showing the number of dioptrics, together with the focal lengths of the series of trial lenses, in the metrical system (worked out to three places of decimals), and in Paris inches,* is given at the end of Snellen's Book of Types.

In the box of trial glasses the lenses are numbered in dioptrics.

---

* A Paris inch is equal to $1\frac{1}{8}$ English inch.

Myopia, M. (*Short sight*).—The antero-posterior axis of the eyeball is of too great a length, so that parallel rays of light are brought to a focus in front of the retina instead of upon it. In order to obviate this we employ concave lenses, which render the parallel rays of light divergent before reaching the cornea, and so remove the point of union, after refraction, further back. The patient complains that he is near-sighted. If test types be given him to read, he will hold them close to the eyes, *but will read the smallest type easily, provided it be held sufficiently near.* If told to look at a distant object, he will very probably screw up his eyelids, so as to narrow the palpebral aperture, and will only be able to make out objects indistinctly, or not at all. Such symptoms should always lead us to suspect myopia.

Myopic persons often complain of spots floating before the eyes (muscæ volitantes). These need cause no anxiety, and we should expect to hear of their existence.

We ascertain the existence of myopia, as well as its degree, by trial with lenses, as follows:—Having placed the patient at 6 metres from the card on which are pasted the letters from

"D = 6" to "D = 60,"* we ask him to try to read them with each eye separately.

Should he be suffering from a high degree of M., he will distinguish none of the letters. We then place the book of small types in the patient's hand and note carefully the greatest distance at which D = 0.5 or D = 0.6 can be made out. We shall generally find that that concave lens, the negative focal length of which corresponds to the greatest distance at which the eye reads distinctly, or a lens a little stronger or weaker than this, will neutralize the myopia. For instance, if in reading the patient holds the types at 20 centimetres, it will be found that a concave lens of 20 centimetres negative focus—*i.e.*, a lens of 5 D—will be about the one which gives the greatest acuteness of vision for distance.

Having ascertained the distance at which the small types can be read, we direct the patient to look again towards the board on which are pasted the types from D = 6 to D = 60, then hold before the eye under examination concave lenses,

* Smaller types, as D = 5, D = 4, D = 3, placed at their proper distances, will do equally well, if we have not a distance of six metres at dispcsal.

beginning with that the focal length of which corresponds to the distance at which the small types were read. We continue the trial *until we have ascertained the weakest concave lens with which the greatest acuteness of vision can be maintained.* We express the degree of M. by the number of dioptrics of this concave lens. For instance, if it is found that a concave lens of —4 D is the weakest with which letters of D=6 can be read at 6 metres, the degree of myopia is expressed as equal to four dioptrics; and we write shortly thus*—R. E., L. E., or B. E., M., 4 D $v = \frac{6}{6}$; if letters of D=6 cannot be read at six metres, but only D=12, D=18, D=36, or even D=60, the degree of myopia may still be expressed by the number of dioptrics of *the weakest concave lens* with which the *greatest possible acuteness of vision* is maintained. In many cases of myopia, especially those of high degree (above 6 D), we find the acuteness of vision has very much diminished. The want of sight is often due to the atrophic changes in the choroid, which are of frequent occurrence in myopia.

---

* R. E., L. E., B. E., abbreviations for right eye, left eye, both eyes; *v*, for acuteness of vision.

We must be careful in testing cases of M. to examine each eye separately, as a great difference is frequently found to exist between them.

Our reasons for finding *the weakest concave lens* is, that we wish only to render the parallel rays of light so divergent that they may reach the retina. If we give a lens which does more than this, the patient will see equally well with it; but as the rays of light are more divergent than is required, they would be brought to a focus behind the retina; he consequently exercises his accommodation in order to overcome the too great divergence, and this we do not desire him to do. *The treatment of myopia* consists in prescribing spectacles or eyeglasses fitted with suitable concave lenses.

In cases of M. of moderate degree (less than 4 D), we give glasses which accurately neutralize the M. to be used for all purposes.

In the higher degrees (greater than 4 D), we shall usually find (excepting in the case of children) that those lenses which accurately neutralize the whole of the M. are too strong for near work. In such cases we may order glasses which neutralize about two-thirds of the M. to be used for all purposes—*i.e.*, in M = 9 D we give lenses of 6 D; these should be worn constantly for some months, after which stronger lenses may be given, *provided they do not make the eyes ache when used for near work.*

If it be necessary that the patient should see at a distance as distinctly as glasses can make him, we may order a pair of double eyeglasses, furnished with lenses which accurately neutralize the M., to be used for looking at distant objects only, whilst spectacles with lenses correcting about two-thirds of the defect are worn for all other purposes.

Persons with slight M. (less than 2 D) need glasses only as a matter of convenience, and require them only for looking at distant objects. We order a double or single eyeglass which accurately neutralizes the M., to be used for this purpose only.

Our great care in prescribing lenses for M. must be, *never to give them too strong.*

Hypermetropia, H. (*Far sight*).—The antero-posterior axis of the eyeball is too short, parallel rays of light are—unless some change in curvature of the dioptric media* take place—brought to a focus behind the retina.

---

* By dioptric media we understand the cornea lens, aqueous and vitreous.

Hypermetropic individuals see well enough at a distance: they can, by exercising the power of accommodation, so increase the curvature of the crystalline lens, that the parallel rays of light are brought accurately to a focus upon the retina.

They can, while young and in good health, and not over-worked—unless the degree of hypermetropia be very high—by still greater tension of accommodation, do the same with the divergent rays of light proceeding from near objects.

Sooner or later, however, the power of accommodation gives out, the double strain can no longer be maintained, and the image of a near object is formed behind the retina instead of upon it.

In order to remedy this condition we give *convex glasses*, which render parallel rays of light convergent before striking the cornea, and so obviate the necessity for the first part of the strain of accommodation, leaving it to be utilized when a near object is looked at.

A patient presents himself complaining that the eyes ache when looking at a near object; that when reading, lines and words—which are at first distinct enough—when looked at for a few minutes run into one another and become misty. He states that if he closes the eyes for a short time, or rubs them, the print again becomes distinct, but soon fades as before; such symptoms should lead us to suspect hypermetropia. In order to diagnose and also to measure the *degree* of hypermetropia by trial with lenses, we place our patient at the distance of 6 metres from the card on which are pasted Snellen's types from D = 6 to D = 60, and ascertain which letters can be read by each eye separately; in other words, we ascertain the "acuteness of vision." We then note down what each eye can do separately, should there be a difference between them; what can be done with both together, should there be no difference.

Thus, suppose that the right eye reads D = 6 at 6 metres, whilst the left eye reads only D = 12, we write R. E. $v. = \frac{6}{6}$, L. E. $v. = \frac{6}{12}$, etc.; should both eyes read D = 6 at 6 metres, or D = 12 at 6 metres, or D = 18 at 6 metres, or whatever the number of the types may happen to be, we write B. E. $v. = \frac{6}{6}$, $\frac{6}{12}$, $\frac{6}{18}$, etc.

Having found a different acuteness of vision in the two eyes, we cover one, and then hold a convex lens of 1 D before the other. Should vision be equally as acute with + 1 D, we try a stronger and still stronger lens, continuing the trial *until the strongest convex lens with which the greatest attainable acuteness of vision can still be maintained has been ascertained.* Having finished one eye, we test the other in the same manner. Should the acuteness of vision in both eyes be equal, we try both together. The number of dioptrics of the strongest convex lens with which the greatest acuteness of vision is maintained, expresses the degree of H. Should the lens be + 4 D, we have a hypermetropia of 4 dioptrics, and so on. The acuteness of vision may be impaired by + 1 D, we then try + 0.75 D or + 0.5 D; should these still cause impairment, we may assume that no H. is present, or that it is what is called latent. *The fact of a person seeing equally as well at a distance through a convex lens as without, certainly indicates H.* The emmetropic eye is rendered artificially myopic by such means, and its acuteness of vision for distant objects is consequently impaired. The strength of the lens found, as described, expresses the degree of what is known as manifest hypermetropia (Hm.); that is, the

H., which corresponds to an amount of accommodative power, which the patient can relax or exert at will. There is always remaining, however, masked by tension of accommodation over which the patient has no control, an amount of H., known as latent hypermetropia (Hl.). In some cases, indeed, as already mentioned, the whole amount of H. may be latent. In old persons, however, whose range of accommodation is but slight, the greater part, if not the whole of the H., will be manifest; in such, distant vision is not only as good with convex lenses as without, but is often very greatly improved by them. If in any case we desire to make out the whole of the H., latent as well as manifest, or to ascertain its existence in a case where we suspect it, but none is manifest, we must paralyze the ciliary muscle, and so destroy the power of accommodation by the installation of a solution of sulphate of atropine (gr. iv to ℥j), used three times a day for two or three days before making the trial.

As a rule, we need only ascertain the manifest hypermetropia. Herein is the necessity for finding the *strongest* convex lens with which the greatest acuteness of vision for distant objects is attainable. We know that in the method we are employing we can only ascertain a part of the existing defect, and our object is to neutralize as much of it as possible.

Having found the strongest convex glass with which the greatest acuteness of vision for distant letters can be attained, we note down its number after the acuteness of vision which we have found to exist without the aid of lenses. Thus, suppose we find B. E. $v. = \frac{6}{6}$, and with + 1 D the same acuteness of vision is still maintained, we note down after B. E. $v. = \frac{6}{6}$ with + 1 D $v. = \frac{6}{6}$, or more shortly B. E. $v. = \frac{6}{6}$ c. + 1 D, $v. = \frac{6}{6}$. If one eye—the right, for instance, have an acuteness of vision $= \frac{6}{12}$, which is improved by the addition of a convex lens, we will suppose it to be + 4 D, and that D = 6—can be read with it, we write R. E. $v. = \frac{6}{12}$ c̄. + 4 D, $v. = \frac{6}{6}$; if it be the left eye, we note in the same manner, substituting L. E. for R. E.; if both eyes, we substitute B. E. for R. E., and so on.

The treatment of hypermetropia consists in prescribing glasses which accurately neutralize the *manifest hypermetropia*, to be used for all near work. Should the symptoms return after such glasses have been worn for a time, we may be sure that too much of the hypermetropia was latent at the time we made our trial, and that the glasses are not strong enough. We repeat the trial, and very probably shall find more manifest hypermetropia; should such be the case, we increase the strength of the glasses in accordance with the result obtained.

Should the trial give the same results as the previous one, we paralyze the accommodation, ascertain the whole hypermetropiá, both manifest and latent, and order glasses which neutralize both.

Astigmatism.—By the term "astigmatism" we understand a condition of asymmetry of the cornea. The asymmetry is of two kinds: in the first there is a difference of curvature between different corneal meridians; in the second there is a difference of curvature in different segments of the same meridian, constituting irregularity. The first form is known as *regular*, the second as *irrègular* astigmatism. The latter defect is frequently complicated by irregular curvature of the crystalline, lens, and in the present state of our knowledge little can be done in the way of treatment. We will therefore dismiss the subject without further notice.

Regular Astigmatism.—A certain amount of regular astigmatism is present in the cornea of the emmetropic eye. Its maximum of curvature (that which has the shortest radius, and consequently the shortest focal length) is found in the vertical meridian; its minimum of curvature (that which has the longest radius, and consequently the longest focal length) is found in the horizontal meridian. If the degree of asymmetry be so slight as to give rise to no impairment of vision, it is known as *normal astigmatism*, or *astigmatism of the normal eye*. But if, on the contrary, defective vision is produced by the asymmetry, it is known as *abnormal astigmatism*.

The existence of normal astigmatism can be very easily demonstrated. If we draw two fine lines on paper, crossing each other at right angles, and look at them in such a position that they correspond to the vertical and horizontal corneal meridians, a distance will be found for every emmetropic eye at which the vertical line can be seen more distinctly than the horizontal, and *vice versa*.

The question at once arises, Why should this difference exist? To answer it, we must understand what are the conditions necessary in order to see a vertical or horizontal line distinctly.

To see a vertical line distinctly, it is requisite that rays of light proceeding from it in a *horizontal direction*, and therefore passing through the horizontal meridian of the cornea, should be brought to a focus in the retina.

To see a horizontal line distinctly, it is necessary that rays of light proceeding from it in a *vertical direction*, and therefore passing through the vertical meridian of the cornea, be brought to a focus in the retina. . As a consequence of this, vertical lines may be considered as belonging to the *horizontal* corneal meridian, and horizontal lines to the *vertical* meridian.

As already stated, the curvature of the cornea has the shortest radius and shortest focal length in its vertical meridian, the longest in its horizontal; consequently it will be found that a fine horizontal line can be *distinctly* seen at a shorter distance than a fine vertical line, a fine vertical line at a somewhat greater distance than a horizontal.

By practising the simple experiment just mentioned, any individual whose eyes are emmetropic can prove to himself the existence of normal astigmatism. What has been said with regard to vertical and horizontal lines applies with equal force to those drawn in any direction. In order to see any line distinctly, rays of light passing through that meridian of the cornea which is at right angles to it must be brought to a focus in the retina. This rule should be borne in mind when working out astigmatism with test lines.

Abnormal astigmatism.—In abnormal astigmatism we find the rule to be that the greatest curvature (that which has the shortest radius) of the cornea is in, or approaching to, the vertical meridian; and the least curvature in or approaching to, the horizontal meridian. The two principal meridians—those of the greatest and least curvature—always stand at right angles to each other.

There are five forms of abnormal astigmatism—in two, one principal meridian of the cornea is normal, that at right angles to it deviating in the direction of too great or too slight curvature; in the first case constituting *simple myopic astigmatism,* in the second *simple hypermetropic astigmatism.* In the third case the whole eye has a myopic refraction, but the curvature of the cornea in one principal meridian is in excess, and consequently the myopia in that meridian increased. This condition is known as *compound myopic astigmatism.* In a fourth the whole eye has a hypermetropic refraction, but the curvature of the cornea in one principal meridian is diminished, and consequently the hypermetropia in that meridian increased. This condition is known as *compound hypermetropic astigmatism.* In a fifth form the curvature of one principal meridian is too great, causing myopia in that meridian; the curvature of the meridian at right angles to it being too slight, and giving rise to hypermetropia. This condition is known as *mixed astigmatism.*

Diagnosis and Treatment.—Such are the conditions which give rise to astigmatism. We have now to consider the methods by which it may be diagnosed and treated.

Whenever in the examination of ametropia by trial with lenses it is found that the acuteness of vision cannot be raised to the normal standard, and that the patient has difficulty in telling which glass suits him best, or states that he sees equally well with two or three of different focal lengths, the existence of astigmatism should be suspected.

A glance with the ophthalmoscope will show that there is no disease of the retina or choroid, opacities of the cornea, lens, or vitreous, etc. The presence of astigmatism can, like that of ametropia, be ascertained by trial with lenses, or by ophthalmoscopic examination.

For the purposes of ascertaining the existence, and also for measuring the degree of astigmatism by trial with lenses, a series of lines radiating from a common centre should be used. A half-circle of such will be found in Dr. Snellen's book of test-types. These we place at a convenient distance (five to six metres), and direct the patient, whose refraction should have been previously tested in the ordinary way, to look towards them. We test each eye separately, and ascertain whether that under examination can distinguish any of the lines without the aid of lenses; if any line can be distinctly seen, its direction should be carefully noted. This at once gives a clue to the form of astigmatism present; and the previous trial of refraction will, in all probability, have furnished evidence of myopia or hypermetropia, although no satisfactory result has been obtained.

Let us suppose that a line running in a vertical or nearly vertical direction is plainly seen; from what has been said respecting the conditions necessary for seeing a vertical line distinctly, we know that the meridian of the cornea situated at right angles to the line which is plainly seen has either a normal or too slight (hypermetropic) curvature. We then direct the patient to keep his eye fixed on this line, and hold a weak convex and concave lens alternately before it; if the line is rendered less distinct by the former of these, and not much altered by the latter, we at once diagnose emmetropia in a meridian approaching the horizontal. Our next care is to ascertain what lens will enable the eye to distinguish a line running at *right angles* to that which is seen without such aid.

The trial should be commenced with that lens, convex or concave, which in the previous trial of refraction was found to give the greatest acuteness of vision: this lens, in the case supposed, will in all probability be a concave one. Such being the case we continue the trial until the weakest concave lens has been found which renders distinct the line standing at right angles to that first seen, whilst the remainder of the half-circle becomes indistinct.

In the case supposed, simple myopic astigmatism is present and its degree is expressed by the number of dioptrics of the weakest concave lens which renders distinct the line running at right angles to that which is most clearly seen without a lens; supposing the lens to be one of 2 D, the degree of astigmatism = 2 D. (Am = 2 D, *i. e.*, myopic astigmatism 2 D.)

In order to check the result obtained, a cylindrical lens* of 2 D should be held before the eye, its axis being at right angles to the line first seen without a spherical glass, and in the same direction as that seen with. If a proper correction has been obtained, the test-line will all appear the same, and the acuteness of vision will be found considerably increased. The other forms of astigmatism are also to be diagnosed by means of the test-lines and trial with lenses.

In simple hypermetropic astigmatism it will generally be found that the horizontal or nearly

---

* Cylindrical lenses are ground upon a cylinder. Only those rays of light passing through such lenses in a direction at right angles to the axis of the cylinder are refracted; those passing in the direction of the axis undergo no change: consequently the cylindrical glass must always be placed with its axis at right angles to that meridian of the cornea on which it is intended to act

horizontal lines are most distinctly seen, and that they are rendered less distinct by the addition of convex lenses, whilst those running at right angles to them are distinguished as easily, or more easily, than before. The trial with lenses should be continued until the *strongest convex lens* has been ascertained, with which the vertical, or nearly vertical, lines can still be distinguished. The degree of astigmatism is expressed by the number of dioptrics of this lens. Supposing the correcting lens to be one of 2 D, then the astigmatism = 2 D. (Ah = 2 D, *i.e.*, hypermetropic astigmatism of 2 D.)

The result obtained must be checked by trial with a convex cylindrical lens, the axis of which must be placed in a more or less vertical direction.

In cases of compound myopic astigmatism, distant vision is generally so imperfect that none of the test-lines can be made out at six metres. Trial with concave lenses, commencing with that which has been previously found, during the trial of refraction, to raise the acuteness of vision most, quickly enables the eye to recognize some of the lines, those situated in a vertical direction being usually first made out. As soon as any line can be recognized, careful trial should be made until the weakest concave lens with which it can still be clearly seen has been ascertained. Having done this, we should next find the weakest concave lens with which a line running in a direction at right angles to that at first seen is clearly made out. The strength of this lens will usually be found to be greater than that of the first. The difference between the two expresses the degree of astigmatism.

Supposing it is found that no lines are made out at first, but that with a lens of 2 D those having a vertical, or nearly vertical, direction are brought clearly into view, and that a lens of 4 D is required to enable the eye under examination to see lines running at right angles to those first distinguished; what do we learn from this result? (1.) That in the horizontal, or nearly horizontal, meridian of the cornea there is myopia of 2 D. (2.) That in a meridian at right angles to this there is myopia of 4 D. To neutralize this we employ a spherical *concave* lens of 2 D: this, of course, corrects 2 D of myopia in all meridians, but we have found by our trial that in one meridian myopia of 4 D exists; consequently, the spherical lens only neutralizes ½ of the defect in this meridian, another 2 D still remaining (4—2=2). In order to correct the remaining myopia, a cylindrical lens of 2 D must be combined with the spherical, the axis of the cylinder being placed in a more or less horizontal direction.

In the case supposed, there is myopia 2 D (M = 2 D), and, besides this, myopic astigmatism 2 D (Am = 2 D). 2 D being the difference between the two meridians.

The result obtained must be checked by testing the acuteness of vision both for lines and letters with a concave spherical lens of 2 D, combined with a concave cylindrical lens also of 2 D.

Compound hypermetropic astigmatism can be diagnosed by the use of lines and trial with lenses in the same manner as the compound myopic, but of course with this difference—that the lenses employed are convex instead of concave. It will generally be found that the eye affected by compound hypermetropic astigmatism has the greatest acuteness of vision for lines running in a more or less horizontal direction, those running in a direction at right angles to these being less distinctly seen.

Having ascertained which of the lines is most distinctly seen, we commence the trial with convex lenses, using first that which was found to give the greatest acuteness of vision during the trial of refraction. The trial must be continued, until the strongest convex lens with which the particular line or lines can still be made out has been ascertained.

Our next care must be to find the strongest convex lens with which lines running at right angles to those at first seen can still be made out.

The strongest lenses, which give the greatest acuteness of vision for lines more or less horizontal and for those having a more or less vertical direction having been ascertained, the degree of astigmatism is expressed by the difference between them. Thus, if lines running in a horizontal direction can still be made out with a convex lens of 2 D, the presence of 2 D of hypermetropia in the vertical meridian of the cornea is demonstrated. If lines running in a vertical direction can be made out through a convex lens of 4 D, there is hypermetropia of 4 D in the horizontal meridian, and the degree of astigmatism is 2 D ($4-2=2$). There is hypermetropia of 2 D in all meridians with an additional 2 D in the horizontal (H = 2 D, Ah = 2 D), *i.e.*, hypermetropia 2 D with hypermetropic astigmatism 2 D. The required correction will be a convex spherical lens of 2 D, combined with a convex cylindrical lens also of 2 D, the axis of the cylinder being placed in a more or less vertical direction.

The correction must be checked by trial of the acuteness of vision for lines and letters when looked at through the above combination of lenses.

The presence of mixed astigmatism can also be diagnosed by ascertaining the acuteness of vision for lines running in different directions, both by trial with lenses and without such aid.

In a case of this form of asymmetry, the eye under examination will probably be found to have a greater power of distinguishing lines which run in a more or less vertical direction than those which have a horizontal inclination, when the half-circle is placed at a distance of 5 to 6 metres.

Let us suppose that on testing an eye, the trial of refraction of which has given no satisfactory result, it is found that lines having a vertical direction are seen with tolerable distinctness. We at once suspect that the meridian at right angles to the lines thus distinguished has a normal or too slight (hypermetropic) curvature. We commence the trial with weak convex lenses: if it is found that vision for the same lines is as acute with these as without, or that the sharpness of sight increases, hypermetropia is certainly present in the horizontal meridian of the cornea. The existence of hypermetropia in the horizontal meridian having been proved, our next care is to ascertain its degree; this is done by finding the strongest convex lenses with which vertical lines can still be distinctly seen; the number of dioptrics of this lens then expresses the degree of hypermetropia. Suppose the lens to be one of 2 D, the degree of hypermetropia in the horizontal meridian is 2 D.

We next proceed to ascertain the refraction in the vertical meridian; it will be found that the convex lenses which did not affect, or even improved, the vision for vertical lines, render horizontal ones still less distinct than before. We then try concave lenses; and if it is found that the vision for horizontal lines is improved, we continue the trial until the weakest concave lens with which the greatest attainable acuteness of vision for horizontal lines is maintained has been ascertained. The number of dioptrics of this lens then expresses the degree of myopia in the vertical meridian. Supposing the lens to be one of 2 D, then the degree of myopia is 2 D; and the eye under examination has, besides hypermetropia of 2 D in the horizontal meridian, myopia of 2 D in the vertical meridian. The degree of astigmatism in this case is the sum of the two, *i. e.*, 4 D. The combination required to neutralize the defect will consist of a convex and a concave cylindrical lens, each of 2 D, placed with their axes at right angles to each other—that of the convex lens being vertical; that of the concave horizontal.

The diagnosis of astigmatism by the ophthalmoscope is very simple. If, on examining an eye by the direct method, it is found that, at a given distance, vessels running over the fundus in one direction are seen (either in an erect or inverted image) more clearly than those having a course more or less at right angles; or that vessels situated in the vertical meridian are seen in an erect position, those situated in the horizontal meridian being seen inverted, astigmatism is present.

The form of asymmetry can be ascertained, according to the rules laid down in the diagnosis of anomalies of refraction by the ophthalmoscope.

Treatment.—The treatment of astigmatism consists in prescribing glasses which neutralize the defect. The optician should be furnished with the number of dioptrics of the required simple cylindrical lens in the case of simple astigmatism; and with that of the required spherical and cylindrical lenses in the case of compound astigmatism: these are combined in one lens, of which one surface is ground to the required spherical curvature, and the opposite surface of the required cylindrical curvature; such a combination is known as a sphericocylindrical lens. We should always see the lenses and test them, and ascertain that their axes are in the proper direction, before they are placed in the permanent frame. Opticians keep frames in which the glasses can be moved, and in which they are sent for approval. In the case of mixed astigmatism, a bicylindrical lens—that is, a lens having one surface ground with a concave cylindrical curvature, the other being made of the requisite convex cylindrical curvature, the axes of the two being placed at right angles to each other—may be ordered. Or, what is preferable, a lens having on one surface a convex spherical curvature may have its opposite surface ground with a concave cylindrical curvature, the strength of this, of course, being increased in proportion as the convex spherical surface increases the myopia in the meridian on which it (the cylindrical lens) is alone intended to act. For instance, in a case where myopia of 2 D exists in the vertical meridian, and hypermetropia 2 D in the horizontal, a lens, one surface of which has a spherical convex curvature of 2 D, may be used; but this, of course, increases the myopia in the vertical meridian by 2 D, consequently the other surface of the glass must be ground with a concave cylindrical surface of 4 D, so as to neutralize the myopia already existing, and that produced by the spherical convex curvature.

In some cases of mixed astigmatism it may be requisite to give glasses which enable the patient to see at a certain definite distance. For instance, in the case supposed above, with myopia 2 D, and hypermetropia 2 D, it might be requisite to bring the farthest point of distinct vision to 50 centimetres, which is the greatest distance at which objects can be distinctly seen through the myopic meridian, and also the negative focal length of the concave lens (2 D), which neutralizes the myopia. This can be accomplished by altering the 2 D of hypermetropia to 2 D of myopia.

Now, a convex cylindrical lens of 2 D neutralizes the hypermetropia, and renders the eye emmetropic in the meridian on which it acts. To induce a myopia of 2 D in this meridian, the curvature of the cylindrical lens must be increased by 2 D; consequently we shall have a convex cylindrical lens of twice 2 D—that is, 4 D; therefore, to make the hypermetropic meridian of 2 D = myopic 2 D, a convex cylindrical lens of 4 D is required.

In working out cases of astigmatism, it will frequently be found that the accommodation continually alters its tension, and with it the focus of the eye under examination. If any very considerable difficulty be experienced from this cause, we shall find it necessary to paralyze the ciliary muscle by the use of a strong solution of atropine (four grains to one ounce), used twice or thrice a day for some few days before the trial with lenses is made.

By *range of accommodation* we understand the power of a lens, which we suppose the crystalline adds to itself, when we change from our farthest to our nearest point of distinct vision. In emmetropia the focal length of this lens equals the distance of the nearest point of distinct vision from the eye.

We determine the range of accommodation thus:—We first ascertain the farthest point of distinct vision by directing our patient to look at distant types. If $D = 6$ can be read at 6 metres, we may suppose the farthest point lies at infinity, the distance being only limited by the size of the object looked at.

We then take the smallest types the patient can read, and see how near they can be brought and still read; this gives us the nearest point of distinct vision.

Let us suppose that the farthest point lies at infinite distance, and the nearest at twenty centimetres; the power of the lens which we suppose the crystalline has added to itself to affect this change is one of $\frac{100}{20} = 5$ D, or five lenses, each of one metre focus, which equals one lens of twenty centimetres focus, the distance from the eye of the nearest point of distinct vision.

Should hypermetropia be present, its degree must be ascertained and added to the range of accommodation determined as above, because the hypermetropic eye is already exercising its accommodative power when adjusted for its far point.

Should myopia be present, its degree must be ascertained and subtracted from the range of accommodation, because the myopic eye sees clearly at a point for which the emmetropic eye has to accommodate.

Presbyopia.

As age advances the range of accommodation becomes less, and the near point recedes from the eye. It has been arbitrarily determined that so soon as the nearest point of distinct vision has receded to beyond 22 cm. from the eye, presbyopia has commenced. We express the degree of presbyopia by the number of dioptrics which are required to bring the near point to 22 cm.

In the emmetropic eye presbyopia may be said to commence after forty years of age; at forty the near point has receded to 22 cm.

The following Table shows the glass required by an emmetropic individual at each period of five years after forty :—

Age	D.
45	1
50	2
55	3
60	4
65	4.5
70	5.5
75	6
80	7

In myopia a glass of less strength will be required, according to the degree of M, thus :— A patient aged fifty, with M of 1 D, instead of requiring a glass of 2 D, will require one of only 1 D, for reading, etc. In cases of myopia above 4.5 D, presbyopia does not occur, as the farthest point of distinct vision is situated at 22 cm. or less, and will recede but little, if at all. In hypermetropia a stronger glass will be required, according to the degree of H, thus :— A patient of fifty, with H of 1 D, will require a convex glass for reading, etc., not of 2 D, but of 3 D. This, however, though theoretically correct, is not found to answer in practice; the patient does not care to have the whole H as well as the presbyopia neutralized. We find it best to prescribe glasses which correct the presbyopia, and about half or two-thirds, not the whole of the H.

SECTION VII.

DISTURBANCE OF VISION—USE OF THE OPHTHALMOSCOPE—NORMAL AND MORBID APPEARANCES.

A PATIENT comes to us complaining of some such defects of sight as the following:—

That he cannot read or do near work for any length of time, but sees fairly well at a distance; that he sees near objects clearly, but can make out nothing distinctly at a distance; that there is a mist before the eyes; that he sees floating bodies or fixed spots; that parts of objects are clearly seen, whilst other parts are obscured; that he can only tell light from dark, or is quite blind.

These symptoms may depend on "anomalies of refraction," already described, opacities of the transparent media of the eye, disease of the structures occupying its fundus, retina, optic nerve, or choroid, or possibly on some affection of the nervous centres.

Should there be no cause for the disturbance of vision, such as dense corneal opacity, advanced cataract, etc., visible to the unaided eye, we ascertain the acuteness and field of vision, test the refraction (*see* Sec. VI.), and having arrived at no satisfactory result, make an examination by lateral illumination and by the ophthalmoscope.*

Examination by Lateral Illumination.—We seat our patient in a dark room, place a lamp in front of him, and rather to his left side, then with a biconvex lens of 16 D (about $2\frac{1}{2}$ inches focal length of the old system) held in the right hand, concentrate the light upon the eye we

---

* The beginner will find his examination much facilitated by dilating the pupil with atropine, and in some cases even an experienced observer may find it impossible to make a satisfactory investigation without such aid; we may either employ a strong solution of sulphate of atropine—gr. ij. or gr. iv. to ℥j of water—which will dilate the pupil in the course of ten minutes or a quarter of an hour, but has the disadvantage that its effects last for some five or six days; or if we are in no hurry, we may order a solution of $\frac{1}{8}$ gr. to ℥j to be used twice or three times in the course of a day, and then make our examination. We should, however, avoid the use of atropine as much as possible, as it may be the cause of a good deal of inconvenience and discomfort to the patient.

wish to examine; by so doing we can diagnose and accurately define morbid changes in cornea, iris, anterior chamber, lens, or anterior portion of vitreous. We shall find that with a little practice each of the above-named structures can be by turns thoroughly illuminated. If we wish to make a very complete examination, we can use a second lens to magnify the parts illuminated by the first. In the normal condition of parts lateral illumination gives chiefly negative results, the cornea appears quite transparent, and the pupil black and clear, or at most a bluish reflection returns from it; or we may make out some radiating lines traversing its area. The bluish reflection is from the crystalline lens, the lines are in the lens, and represent the planes of junction of the various bundles of fibres which make up its substance—sectors of the lens, as they are sometimes called. The morbid changes that we shall most commonly meet with are corneal opacities, opacities upon the lens capsule, the latter occurring as white dots, or streaks, or as dark spots, consisting of uvea detached from the posterior surface of the iris; adhesions of the iris to the lens capsule ("posterior synechiæ") of varying extent, at times only a few tags existing, at others the whole of the margin of the pupil being firmly bound down, whilst its area is blocked by opaque material; opacities in the lens itself (cataract), either central, peripheral, situated at its anterior or posterior poles, or involving its whole substance, and occasionally a growth or blood-clot occupying the anterior portion of the vitreous chamber.

Examination by the Ophthalmoscope.

Direct Method, or Examination of the Erect Image.—In this method of examination we use the mirror alone, and we see what is known as a virtual image,* which is erect in position, and in reality situated behind the eye. We conduct the examination thus:—Having seated our patient as for lateral illumination, we place a lamp at the side corresponding to the eye to be examined, on a level with, but so situated as to leave the cornea in shade; we then direct him to look forwards and a little upwards, and keep the eyes as steady as possible. We will now sup-

* See Ganot's "Elementary Physics," ninth edition, p. 394, or any other similar work.

pose that we wish to examine the right eye, and have placed the patient and lamp as directed; we stand opposite, a distance of eighteen inches or two feet separating our own from the observed eye, take the ophthalmoscope in the right hand, look through the sight-hole with the right eye, and reflect the light from the lamp into the pupil of the patient's right eye. If the examination be properly conducted, we shall see that the pupil, instead of appearing black, returns a bright red reflection. We next look for the optic disc, which lies somewhat to the inner side of the axis of the eyeball. We know when we are looking at the disc from the alteration in color of the reflection through the pupil, which changes from bright red to white or pink. Having obtained the reflection peculiar to the optic disc, we approach until an interval of only two inches separates our own cornea from that of the observed eye. Having approached thus near, supposing that both our own and the observed eye are emmetropic, and that the accommodation of both be relaxed, we shall see a distinct erect and considerably magnified image of the optic disc and retinal vessels; we should examine all parts of the interior of the globe by looking in different directions through the pupil.

The examination of the erect image requires much more practice than that of the inverted, but we should all try to become proficient in it, as we can by its aid make out minute changes in the fundus of the eye much more accurately than by examination of the inverted image alone.

It is useless our trying to examine the erect image in an eye which is myopic, or if we suffer from myopia ourselves, unless we first place behind the sight-hole of the ophthalmoscope a concave lens which will neutralize the myopia in either case. Should both the eye we wish to examine and our own be myopic, we must use a lens sufficiently strong to neutralize the defect in both, or we may place a lens which corrects the myopia of the observed eye behind the sight-hole of the ophthalmoscope, and wear the spectacles or other glasses we are in the habit of using for looking at distant objects.

If we wish to examine the patient's left eye, we use our own left eye, hold the mirror in the left hand, and place the lamp at the patient's left side.

By the direct method of examination we can make out the same morbid changes as seen by lateral illumination, but opacities instead of appearing of their proper color (white, brown, etc.), are dark, and situated on the red background formed by the reflection from the fundus of the eye.

We also discover opacities in the vitreous. These are seen as dark or greyish spots, threads, or clouds, usually floating about as the eye is moved. The dark opacities are often the result of hæmorrhage, the grey ones of inflammation.

Displacements of the retina, appearing as a bluish grey movable cloud, occupying some part (the lower by preference) of the fundus of the eye. The cloud is seen to jerk up and down, as the eyeball is moved; the retinal bloodvessels can in most cases be traced over its surface. The displacement may vary in size from slight wrinkling of a small portion to separation of the whole retina from the choroid, the only points of attachment remaining being at the optic disc and ciliary processes. We can also ascertain the condition of refraction; thus supposing we make out *clearly* the details of a bloodvessel, portion of the optic disc, or other object occupying the fundus of the examined eye, whilst still separated from it by a considerable interval, we may be sure that we are dealing with some anomaly of refraction.

We determine the nature of anomaly present by ascertaining the position of the image we see; it may be inverted or erect; if the former, we are dealing with a case of myopia, if the latter, with one of hypermetropia.

The position of the image may be ascertained by either of the following methods. First having plainly distinguished some object, a bloodvessel, for instance, we steadily approach the observed eye, taking care the while to direct the light properly, and keep the object in view. If as the observed eye is approached we find that the object becomes indistinct and at length fades entirely from view, the image is a real or inverted one, the retina lies beyond the focus of the cornea lens and humors (dioptric system, as they are called), and the eye is myopic. If, on the contrary, as we approach the object retains its distinctness, or becomes even more plainly visible, the retina lies within the focus of the dioptric system, the image is virtual or erect, and the eye is hypermetropic. As previously stated, we can make out nothing of the details of the emmetropic eye until we have approached to within two inches of it. The second test is:—Having obtained a distinct image of a retinal bloodvessel, we direct the patient to keep his eye fixed on some suitably situated object, then move our own head from side to side; should the image be inverted it will move in an opposite, should it be erect in the same, direction as our head.

Indirect Method, or Examination of the Inverted Image.—In this method of examination we use the mirror, aided by a biconvex lens, and we see what is known as a real image.* The image is inverted and is situated in the air between our eye and the biconvex lens.

The preliminary steps in the examination of the inverted image are the same as for that of the erect image, we may, however, keep the lamp on the same side in the examination of either eye.

We will again suppose that we wish to examine the right eye; having obtained the red reflection we do not approach, but remain at a distance of eighteen inches, and direct the patient

* See Ganot's "Elementary Physics," ninth edition, p 393.

to look at some object so situated that the axis of the observed eye is turned somewhat inwards. We then hold a biconvex lens of two and a half or three inches (16 or 13 D) focal length in front of the eye, at a distance about equal to its focal length from the cornea, steadying it by placing the ring and little fingers upon the patient's brow.

Thus an inverted image of the optic disc and retinal vessels is formed, which although apparently within the eye, is in reality situated in the air between the observer and the biconvex lens.

We must remember that the distance of the image from our eye is much less than it appears to be, and consequently in order to see it distinctly we must put our accommodation more or less upon the stretch, as in looking at any other near object. We shall, however, find the examination much facilitated by habitually using behind the sight-hole of the ophthalmoscope a convex lens of twelve inches focal length (old system) 3.5 D of the new. This enables us to see the image extremely well defined, and somewhat magnified, provided that it be not situated at a greater distance than twelve inches (28 centimetres) from our eye, and this without tension of accommodation. As in the examination of the erect image, we should use our right eye in the examination of the patient's right eye, and our left in the examination of the left.

Having examined the optic disc and retina immediately surrounding we direct the patient to look straight at the mirror, this brings the region of the yellow spot—the central and most sensitive part of the retina—into view; we then direct him to look upwards, downwards, to the right, and left, and thus in turn examine all the more peripheral parts of the fundus.

Normal Appearance of Parts seen by the Ophthalmoscope.

The retina is either quite transparent and colorless, or in dark eyes may appear as a faintly grey cloud, covering the choroid. Its position is marked by that of its bloodvessels. The bright red reflection, which is so striking, is due to the blood in the choroid. The depth of color of the reflection varies with the amount of pigmentation; in blue or grey eyes it is light red, in dark ones of a much deeper tint, and in the negro appears dark blue.

The parts of the fundus oculi requiring special attention are the optic disc and parts immediately surrounding it, and the region of the yellow spot.

The disc appears, at first sight, to be of a uniform pink color, but on closer examination different parts are found to present different shades.

Its centre is pale, or even white; next succeeds a zone of pink, this being again bounded by an apparently double border of lighter color. The pale appearance of the centre of the disc is caused by connective tissue surrounding the bloodvessels. The succeeding pink zone consists entirely of nerve fibres and delicate capillaries. The outer pale double border is formed by the sclerotic and choroidal rings, which do not accurately cover each other, the choroidal ring being of somewhat greater diameter than the sclerotic opening, the margin of which, being left uncovered by pigment, shines through the transparent nerve fibres.

Both the white central portion and the outer ring may be, in some cases, so distinctly marked as to lead us to mistake them for morbid appearance; but both conditions are perfectly consistent with health. From the pale central portion of the disc proceed the bloodvessels of the retina; these usually appear upon the nerve surface at the same point, but may emerge separately or in groups of two or three.

The vessels usually divide into about eight principal branches upon the surface of the disc or in the retina near its margin. Four of these are arteries, the remaining four veins; two of each pass upwards, and a like number downwards, to be distributed over the retina. The lateral branches are insignificant, and are given off from the principal trunks near the margin of the disc.

The veins are distinguished from the arteries by their greater calibre (the proportion being about as three to two), their darker color, and by the fact that the arteries are marked by a double contour, their margins being considerably darker than their centres.

Certain phenomena are not unfrequently observed with the ophthalmoscope, which, although contrary to the general rule, are perfectly consistent with health.

We may make out a network of pale pink bands. These are the choroidal vessels, which in light eyes often show very plainly.

Occasionally a dark spot is seen in one of the larger bloodvessels at its commencement or termination in the disc. This is caused by a peculiar arrangement of the vessel which is passing backwards through the transparent nerve fibres, and is seen on end.

Spontaneous pulsation of the retinal veins may be met with. It is, however—unlike spontaneous arterial pulsation—perfectly consistent with health. (*See* Glaucoma, Sec. III.)

A dark crescentic figure bordering some part of the margin of the disc is caused by an accumulation of pigment, and is congenital.

An appearance of wisp-like patches of brilliant white, bordering some part of the disc, and extending for a variable distance into the surrounding retina, obscuring the vessels in parts, and at times continuing along their borders in the form of white threads, is also congenital, and caused by a continuation of the opaque nerve sheaths, which should end at the lamina cribrosa, into the retina.

We may meet with excavation of the central portion of the optic disc—"physiological cup," as it is called. We find the white central portion of the disc, already alluded to, extremely well defined and enlarged, the vessels upon its surface being twisted in a peculiar manner. If when employing the indirect method of examination we move the biconvex lens from side to side, we shall see that the trunks of the vessels at the bottom of the depression make wider excursions than the branches which lie at the level of the retina. The physiological pit extends nearer to the outer than the inner margin of the disc. As age advances the refractive media become less transparent, the retina grows somewhat hazy, and the disc becomes somewhat paler.

The region of the yellow spot presents in health no very marked ophthalmoscopic appearances, but requires to be carefully examined, as it is very frequently the seat of pathological changes. The yellow spot is the central and most sensitive part of the retina: with the ophthalmoscope, however, we discover nothing yellow about it. Its position is marked by the absence of bloodvessels, which appear to avoid this part, passing above and below it; by some deepening in color, and in some cases a dark, ill-defined oval figure, the long axis of which is horizontal, can be made out.

Every ophthalmoscopic examination should be made upon a certain definite plan. We should first ascertain the condition of the refractive media by lateral illumination; second, ascertain the state of refraction and of the vitreous chamber by direct ophthalmoscopic examination; third, take a general survey of the fundus by the indirect method; and fourth, having discovered any morbid change, we should work it out carefully by the direct method.

Morbid Appearances.

The diseased conditions most commonly met with are inflammation of the optic disc (optic neuritis, neuro retinitis); the optic disc and retina immediately surrounding are grey, opaque, swollen, and blood-stained. The retinal veins are somewhat enlarged and tortuous, the arteries being narrower than normal; the number of vessels visible is less than in health, and many of those that can be seen are concealed in parts of their course by the opaque material in the optic nerve and retina, so that they appear as parts of bloodvessels broken off.

Congestion of the optic disc (choked disc, "ischæmia"); the disc is red, resembling the surrounding choroid in color, greatly swollen, as shown by projection into the vitreous chamber and increase in area; its transparency is, however, unaffected; its margin is marked by a peculiar bend in the retinal vessels, the retina immediately surrounding the disc is somewhat œdematous and swollen. The retinal veins are enormously distended, the arteries are of about their normal calibre; the number of vessels visible is increased; none of the vessels are concealed from view in any part of their course, but some of them may appear darker or lighter, according as they lie near the surface, or deeply in the œdematous portion of the retina.

In ischæmia, as in neuritis, hæmorrhages may exist on the surface of the disc, or in the surrounding retina.

We seldom see "ischæmia" among the ophthalmic cases, as it causes little or no impairment of vision; it is, however, common enough in the medical wards.

Treatment.—Both optic neuritis and "ischæmia" usually affect both eyes, and indicate disease within the skull; in many cases treatment is of no avail; we should, however, act upon the supposition that there is something or other which may be absorbed, and prescribe accordingly. We may lay it down as a broad rule that the existence of optic neuritis, or "ischæmia," calls for the administration of iodide of potassium, and plenty of it.

Inflammation of the retina, "retinitis," is usually the result of some general condition, syphilis or Bright's disease, against which treatment must be directed.

We find some part of the fundus occupied by opacity, which conceals or obscures the retinal vessels. The opacity may be only a diffused cloudiness, or we may find dense white or grey patches, some of which have a peculiar glistening appearance; blood spots are of frequent occurrence.

A form of degeneration of the retina, which gives most striking ophthalmoscopic appearances, is known as "retinitis pigmentosa." We find spots and patches of black pigment distributed about the retina, most thickly in its peripheral parts, and along the course of its bloodvessels. The optic disc is pale and the retinal bloodvessels are diminished in calibre and visible number. Along with these appearances we find peculiar visual phenomena, the patient becomes blind as the light begins to fail (night blindness), and his field of vision gradually contracts.

Hæmorrhage may occur in the retina independently of retinitis; we may find one or more patches of blood usually in the course of one of the vessels, there may be a slight halo of dulness around the effused blood. The blood may become entirely absorbed, or as time goes on degenerative changes may set in, the clot becomes mottled, and is at length left as a dirty white patch, around which is collected more or less dark pigment.

Inflammation of the choroid, "choroiditis," like inflammation of the retina, usually depends on some constitutional cause, syphilis being by far the most common.

Choroiditis is characterized by the presence of yellowish patches or spots situated in the choroid; when several spots exist scattered about the fundus, we speak of the disease as "choroiditis deseminata." We know that the yellow patches or spots are in the choroid, by noticing that the retinal vessels lie in front of, and are unobscured by them. The yellow exudation will eventually become absorbed, but very frequently leaves evidence of its former existence in patches of atrophy. We see the atrophic patches as white, or dirty white figures, the margins of which are often dark. The whiteness is caused by the destruction of the choroidal pigment and bloodvessels, allowing the sclerotic to come more or less plainly into view; the dark margins are caused by accumulation of pigment.

One form of atrophic change in the choroid which—although very probably of inflammatory origin—does not depend on constitutional causes, is met with in myopic eyes. We see it as a white more or less crescentic figure bordering the outer margin of the optic disc, we often describe it as the crescent of myopia or as posterior staphyloma. The tunics of the eyeball corresponding to the white figure are bulged backwards; the size of the crescent bears a direct ratio to the degree of myopia.

Treatment.—In retinitis—except it be associated with albuminuria or in retinitis pigmentosa—and also in choroiditis, we should give mercurials, so as to hasten the absorption of the already effused material, and prevent more being poured out. We should shield the eyes from light by a shade or protectors, and give rest to the ciliary muscle and iris by paralysing them with atropine.

When atrophy of the choroid has set in, no treatment is of much avail. We can, however, prevent the increase of the atrophic crescent in myopia by prescribing proper spectacles.

Retinitis pigmentosa and retinitis albuminuria should be treated by tonics, none being better than the perchloride of iron. The former, however, leads almost certainly to blindness, in spite of treatment, but it may be many years before vision is completely destroyed.

Atrophy of the optic disc may follow optic neuritis, when it is called consecutive atrophy, or may come on gradually without any previous inflammatory stage, progressive or simple atrophy; vision is reduced to perception of light. The disc is changed in color; in place of its natural pink we find it white, or bluish white. Should the atrophy have followed neuritis, we may find the margins of the disc irregular, in consequence of the previous swelling, but in simple atrophy its edge is always well defined;

the disc may appear shrunken, and at times cupped. Atrophy of the retina occurs under much the same conditions as, and is generally associated with, atrophy of the optic nerve. The retinal vessels become extremely thin, and their visible number is decreased; we may find opaque spots or patches in different parts of the retina.

Treatment.—The treatment of atrophic changes in the optic nerve and retina is hopeless. We should, however, do our best to improve our patient's general health, and give him whatever encouragement we can; thus, should some vision remain, and no change have taken place for some months, we may confidently predict that there will be no further failure of sight.

SECTION VIII.

INJURIES.

Wounds of the eyelids, however extensive or ragged, should be thoroughly cleansed and brought accurately together by any number of sutures that may be required; they will usually heal by primary union.

Ecchymosis of the lids (black eye) is of very frequent occurrence. It needs no treatment; but should it be desired to get quickly rid of the effused blood, the application of a poultice made of equal parts of the scraped root of black bryony and bread crumbs will cause very rapid absorption. The poultice gives rise to a good deal of stinging pain, but must be kept on as long as the patient can bear it.

Emphysema of the lids may occur from rupture of the mucous membrane of the nose, air being forced into the cellular tissue of the eyelids on sneezing or making any violent expiratory effort. Gentle pressure with cotton wool and a bandage, violent expiratory efforts, as blowing the nose, etc., being avoided for the time, will cause the removal of the air.

In any case of increased vascularity of the conjunctiva which has come on suddenly, without apparent cause, and more especially if one eye only be affected, we should suspect the presence of a foreign body. As a rule, patients tell us they have got something in the eye, but now and again they do not know of anything of the sort. Such cases are frequently treated for weeks as ophthalmia, and without benefit.

The foreign body may be found upon the surface of the palpebral conjunctiva, in the fornix, lying on the caruncle, or upon some part of the ocular conjunctiva; but the most frequent situation is just within the margin of the upper lid. Foreign bodies must be removed. If they lie upon the surface of the conjunctiva they can be easily taken away with a spill of paper, any small blunt instrument, such as a pencil, or with the finger-nail.

A foreign body sometimes becomes imbedded in the conjunctiva, when its removal is by no means so easy as we might expect. We must fix the eyelids open with a speculum, cut through the conjunctiva over the foreign body with scissors, and remove it with the point of a knife, or with forceps. Should the patient be unsteady we must employ an anaesthetic. A foreign body, when situated in the most frequent position (just within the margin of the upper lid), is often removed without our knowledge while everting the lid. Should this happen, our examination gives a negative result, but the patient expresses himself relieved.

After removal of the offending substance the vascularity quickly subsides; no after-treatment beyond bathing with warm water is required. The conjunctiva may be cut or torn; such wounds heal readily enough. Should a large gap have been made, the edges must be brought together with a suture, otherwise the application of a pad of lint and bandage for a few days is sufficient.

Burns are usually caused by contact with lime or hot metals; the damage done may be but slight, or the whole conjunctiva and cornea may be converted into a dead white slough.

The conjunctiva must be carefully examined, and all foreign bodies and portions of sloughy tissue removed; should the injury have been caused by lime the conjunctiva must be carefully cleansed with a weak solution of acetic acid, or with simple warm water, a drop of solution of atropine (gr. iv to ℥j) placed between the lids, and the eye carefully bound up with wet lint and a bandage. Should there be much discharge the eye should be bathed with alum lotion three or four times a day. In any case atropine should be dropped in occasionally, so as to keep the pupil well dilated. When the sloughs separate care must be taken to prevent adhesion between the raw surfaces by passing a probe between them daily, and directing the patient to draw the lids away from the globe frequently.

A plastic operation will very probably be needed at some later period.

Hæmorrhage into the substance of the conjunctiva may occur spontaneously or from injury; no treatment is needed.

Simple abrasions of the cornea, if not complicated by the presence of a foreign body, pieces of grit, steel, etc., need only that a drop of solution of atropine be placed between the lids, and the eye bound up with lint and a bandage; they will heal in the course of a few days, but are frequently exquisitely painful at first.

Should a foreign body be lodged in the cornea it must be removed in the following manner:—We place the patient in a chair and stand behind him in the same position as for slitting the canaliculus, keep the lids well open with the fore and middle fingers of the left hand, and steady the eyeball as much as possible by pressing the forefinger (which should hold the upper lid) lightly backwards between the margin of the orbit and the globe, then with the point of a penknife, cataract knife, or small spud made for the purpose, held in the right hand, gently lift the foreign body from its bed; this will not be done as easily as might be imagined, especially if the piece of steel, grit, or whatever it may happen to be, is deeply imbedded in the cornea. Having removed the foreign body, we place some oil and a drop of atropine between the lids, and order the eye to be kept bound up. If any symptoms of iritis or corneitis set in, these must be treated.

Perforating wounds of the cornea generally involve the iris or lens, or both; some prolapse of the iris through the wound will generally have taken place, and not unfrequently the lens will be found becoming more or less opaque, traumatic cataract—we order the eye to be bathed frequently with belladonna lotion, and to be kept bound up with a piece of lint soaked in the same placed over the closed lids; if there be much pain we order two or three leeches to the corresponding temple. These cases generally require some operative interference at a later period. More extensive wounds of the eyeball, especially if passing through the ciliary region, must always be looked upon with suspicion, and watched with the greatest care; as long as there is good perception of light, and no particular pain, we treat them in the same manner as perforating wounds of the cornea; but should the pain increase and all sight be lost, excision of the eyeball will most likely have to be performed, nevertheless should the eye still see light excision must not be done till absolutely necessary; if the injured eye be quite blind or there be any irritation of its fellow, even though the injured one still retain perception of light, the sooner the injured eyeball is removed the better. Cases of smash of the globe require instant removal of its remains.

www.ingramcontent.com/pod-product-compliance
Lightning Source LLC
Chambersburg PA
CBHW030539270326
41927CB00008B/1438
* 9 7 8 3 3 3 7 8 1 5 4 7 9 *